M.C. SAIBO

The Healing Embrace of Nature

Discovering Wellness: Unleashing the Healing Power of Nature in Your Life

Contents

1

Introduction

1.Introduction

A. Definition of Nature Healing

In the quiet spaces where leaves rustle, birdsong hums, and the earth breathes, there exists an undeniable force - the healing touch of nature. Nature healing, as I explore in this journey through words and wonder, is not a prescription, but an ancient remedy for the afflictions that ail our modern souls. It is the soothing balm that mends our minds, the gentle breeze that whispers peace to our hearts.

B. Importance of Embracing Nature for Well-being

In the relentless pace of our modern lives, we often forget the profound connection between our well-being and the natural world. The concrete jungles we've constructed around us may provide convenience, but they seldom offer solace. As we delve into the importance of embracing nature for our well-being, we begin to unravel the intricate dance between our existence and the rhythm of the natural world.

To understand this connection is to acknowledge that we are not isolated beings, but integral threads woven into the vast tapestry of the Earth. The trees, the rivers, the mountains - they are not mere background scenery but essential partners in our journey towards a healthier, more harmonious life.

C. Overview of the Book

This book is an odyssey into the heart of nature healing, a pilgrimage where we rediscover the wisdom embedded in the landscapes that surround us. It is an invitation to pause, breathe, and embrace the world outside our windows, for therein lies the essence of our well-being.

As we traverse the pages ahead, we will wander through enchanted forests, traverse serene meadows, and linger by babbling brooks. Each chapter is a stepping stone, guiding us deeper into the intricate labyrinth of nature's therapeutic embrace. From the secrets whispered by ancient trees to the healing touch of a sun-kissed breeze, we shall uncover the transformative power of nature.

2. The Symphony of Trees

A. The Whispers of Ancient Wisdom

Our journey commences amidst the grandeur of ancient trees, their towering forms carrying the weight of centuries. In the cool shade beneath their branches, we discover a timeless symphony - the whispers of ancient wisdom. It is here that nature reveals its first secret: the art of resilience. Like the trees that weather storms and stand tall despite adversity, we too can find strength in our roots.

As we walk amongst the giants, we learn to listen, not just with our ears but with our hearts. The language of the forest is subtle, a dialect of rustling leaves and creaking branches. To embrace nature healing is to decipher this silent conversation, understanding that within its rhythm lies the key to unlocking our inner peace.

B. The Dance of Light and Shadow

In the heart of the forest, where sunlight filters through the foliage, we encounter the dance of light and shadow. It is a spectacle that mirrors the ebb and flow of life itself. Nature teaches us that shadows are not ominous, but integral to the beauty of existence. Within the interplay of light and darkness, we discover balance and acceptance.

As we immerse ourselves in this dappled realm, we begin to understand that embracing nature is not just about basking in the light but finding grace in the shadows. It is a journey towards self-discovery, where we learn to appreciate the mosaic of our own complexities, just as the forest celebrates both sunlight and shade.

3. *The Serenity of Flowing Waters*

A. The Therapeutic Murmurs

Our pilgrimage now leads us to the banks of a meandering river, where the therapeutic murmurs of flowing waters invite us into a world of serenity. The rhythm of the river is a gentle reminder that life, like its currents, is in constant motion. To embrace nature healing is to understand the art of going with the flow, allowing the waters of change to shape our course.

Beside the river, we shed the burdens of yesterday and embrace the promise of tomorrow. The soothing melody of flowing waters becomes a lullaby, cradling us into a state of tranquility. In this chapter of our exploration, we learn that the river of life, with all its twists and turns, is a source of renewal and rejuvenation.

B. The Reflective Pools of Stillness

Further downstream, we encounter reflective pools that mirror the surrounding landscape with a crystal-clear precision. Here, nature whispers another lesson - the art of stillness. As we gaze into the mirror-like waters, we learn that true reflection comes not in constant movement, but in the quiet moments of contemplation.

Embracing nature is an invitation to create these reflective pools within ourselves, to find moments of stillness amidst life's turbulence. In the depths of contemplative waters, we discover the clarity to navigate the currents of our own existence.

4. The Wisdom of Open Meadows

A. The Canvas of Possibility

Our journey now leads us to expansive meadows, where the open sky stretches above like a vast canvas of possibility. In the embrace of these open spaces, we learn the wisdom of expansiveness. Nature healing unfolds in the freedom of open meadows, where the boundaries of our thoughts and dreams can expand limitlessly.

In the meadows, the wind carries the whispers of untold stories, encouraging us to explore the horizons of our own narratives. To embrace nature is to acknowledge that, like the meadows, our minds too can be boundless fields of potential waiting to be explored.

B. The Dance of Wildflowers

Among the open meadows, we encounter the dance of wildflowers, an intricate ballet of colors and fragrances. In this chapter, we explore the interconnectedness of all living things, discovering that our well-being is intricately linked to the well-being of the world around us. Just as the wildflowers rely on the sun, soil, and rain, we too thrive when nurtured by the elements of a harmonious existence.

As we wander through these floral tapestries, we realize that to embrace nature healing is to recognize the delicate dance of interconnectedness, where our own well-being is entwined with the flourishing vitality of the Earth.

5. Conclusion

In the concluding pages of this chapter, we find ourselves at the intersection of ancient trees, flowing waters, and open meadows.

Nature healing, as we have discovered, is not a linear journey but a mosaic of experiences, each revealing a facet of the profound connection between our well-being and the natural world.

As we step back from this exploration, we carry with us the wisdom of the forest, the serenity of flowing waters, and the expansiveness of open meadows. The embrace of nature, we realize, is not a destination but an ongoing journey, an ever-unfolding narrative that beckons us to return to the heart of healing.

May we, like the trees that stand resilient in the face of storms, find strength in our roots. May we, like the flowing river, navigate the currents of change with grace. And may we, like the open meadows, embrace the boundless possibilities that lie within the expansive landscapes of our own souls.

In the chapters that follow, we will delve even deeper into the tapestry of nature healing, exploring the nuances of each element that beckons us towards a more profound connection with the world outside our windows. For now, let us linger in the echo of rustling leaves, the murmur of flowing waters, and the dance of wildflowers, for therein lies the healing embrace of nature.

2

Nature's Healing Tapestry

A. Scientific Basis of Nature's Therapeutic Effects

In the intricate dance between science and the natural world, we discover the profound symphony of healing that nature orchestrates. At the heart of this melody lies a compelling truth – the scientific basis of nature's therapeutic effects. As we embark on this exploration, we peel back the layers of empirical evidence that reveal how the rustle of leaves and the scent of earth contribute to our well-being.

Science, in its pursuit of understanding, has delved into the intricate mechanisms that make nature a potent elixir for the human soul. The calming effects of natural environments on our nervous system, the reduction of stress hormones in response to the great outdoors – these are not merely poetic notions but verifiable phenomena. We find ourselves drawn into the embrace of green spaces, not just for aesthetic pleasure, but as a prescription for our mental and physical health.

B. Historical Perspectives on Nature as a Healer

As we journey through the pages of time, we encounter a tapestry woven with threads of nature's healing touch. Historical perspectives on nature as a healer reveal a timeless relationship between humanity and the natural world. From the therapeutic gardens of ancient civilizations to the sanatoriums nestled in the embrace of mountain landscapes, our ancestors intuitively understood the remedial power of nature.

In the Renaissance, physicians prescribed the healing airs of the countryside to rejuvenate both body and spirit. In the 19th century, the emergence of the picturesque landscape movement reflected not only an artistic inclination but a recognition of nature's ability to restore balance to the human soul. These echoes from the past resonate in our present, urging us to reconnect with the healing traditions that have shaped our collective understanding of nature.

C. Case Studies Highlighting Positive Health Outcomes

The stories of individuals who have experienced transformative health outcomes through nature's embrace weave a compelling narrative of hope and healing. Case studies become windows into the tangible impact that nature has on our physical and mental well-being.

In the quiet corners of healthcare institutions, we encounter the pioneering efforts to integrate nature into the healing process. From hospital gardens designed to provide respite for patients to nature-based therapies for mental health disorders, these case studies illuminate the potential for positive health outcomes when nature becomes an integral part of our healing environments.

One such story unfolds in the heart of an urban landscape, where a community park becomes a sanctuary for individuals facing chronic health challenges. Through meticulously designed green spaces, the residents discover a haven where the rhythms of nature synchronize with the rhythms of their own healing journeys. The evidence is not just anecdotal; it is a testament to the measurable improvements in physiological markers and overall well-being.

In another case, we journey to the serene landscapes of rural retreats where individuals with stress-related ailments find solace amidst the simplicity of nature. The measurable reduction in cortisol levels and the improvement in sleep patterns tell a story of nature's quiet yet potent ability to restore the delicate balance between health and harmony.

Through these case studies, we witness the alchemy that occurs when individuals are enveloped in the healing embrace of nature. It is a reminder that our connection to the natural world is not just a whimsical notion but a crucial component of the healing journey.

As we navigate the nexus between science, history, and individual narratives, the overarching theme emerges – nature is not merely a backdrop to our lives; it is an active participant in our well-being. In the chapters to come, we will delve deeper into the canvas of nature's healing tapestry, exploring the myriad ways in which the natural world shapes our physical, mental, and emotional health. For now, let us linger in the profound truth that has transcended centuries and scientific paradigms alike – nature, in all its complexity, is an unparalleled healer.

3

Embracing Nature's Presence

A. Building a Personal Connection

In the quietude of a forest, where sunlight filters through the leaves like a cascade of golden memories, we find the first step in our journey toward well-being – building a personal connection with nature. This connection is not a mere acquaintance; it is a dance of reciprocity between our hearts and the world outside.

As we step onto the path that winds through the ancient grove, we are invited to engage our senses fully. The texture of the bark beneath our fingertips, the earthy scent rising from the soil, the symphony of bird calls overhead – these are the threads that weave the fabric of our connection. Building a personal relationship with nature is an intimate process, a conversation in which we listen as much as we speak.

In the embrace of a favorite tree or the warmth of a sunlit meadow, we discover that this connection is not reserved for the chosen few. It is a birthright, waiting to be claimed by those willing to slow down and engage in a dialogue with the natural world. Through this dialogue, we find not only solace but a profound understanding that we are part of something much larger than ourselves.

B. Mindfulness Practices in Natural Settings

As we traverse deeper into the heart of our connection with nature, we encounter the art of mindfulness – a practice that transforms a simple walk in the woods into a sacred pilgrimage. Mindfulness in natural settings is not about escaping the present moment; it is about fully inhabiting it.

In the gentle rustle of leaves and the rhythmic cadence of a babbling brook, we discover the anchors for our awareness. Each step becomes a meditation, each breath an invitation to be present. The forest becomes a cathedral of mindfulness, where the worries of yesterday and the uncertainties of tomorrow dissolve into the dappled sunlight filtering through the leaves.

The practice of mindfulness in nature is a conscious surrender to the moment, an acknowledgment that our well-being is intricately tied to our ability to be fully present. In this chapter of our exploration, we learn that the therapeutic effects of nature are not passive; they are activated through our intentional engagement with the world around us.

C. Cultivating a Sense of Awe and Wonder

Amidst the towering trees and expansive landscapes, we find the gateway to a profound emotional experience – cultivating a sense of awe and wonder. Nature, in all its complexity and beauty, has the power to evoke a feeling of reverence that transcends the boundaries of the ordinary.

As we gaze at a star-studded sky or witness the birth of a sunrise, we are humbled by the grandeur of the natural world. Awe, in its essence, is the recognition of something greater than ourselves. It is the bridge between the finite and the infinite, the moment when our hearts expand to accommodate the vastness of the universe.

In the embrace of awe, we find a balm for the soul. Scientifically, the experience of awe has been linked to reduced stress levels and an increased sense of well-being. But beyond the scientific correlations, awe is a reminder that we are but small players in a grand cosmic narrative.

To cultivate a sense of awe and wonder is to rekindle the childlike curiosity that resides within us. It is an invitation to explore the world with wide-eyed appreciation, to marvel at the intricacies of a dew-kissed spider web or the dance of fireflies on a summer night.

In the chapters to follow, we will delve even deeper into the art of connecting with nature, exploring the nuances of this profound relationship. But for now, let us linger in the stillness of a sun-dappled glade, practicing mindfulness and cultivating awe. For in these moments of connection, we find not only the healing touch of nature but a pathway to a richer, more meaningful existence.

4

Unraveling the Threads of Stress: Nature's Soothing Symphony

A. Impact of Nature on Stress Hormones

In the quiet communion between our bodies and the natural world, a delicate ballet unfolds - the impact of nature on stress hormones. As we navigate the intricacies of modern life, stress often becomes an unwelcome companion, infiltrating our minds and bodies with its demanding presence. Yet, amidst the chaos, nature stands as a steadfast ally, offering a respite that science confirms and the soul intuitively craves.

Research, like a gentle breeze through the leaves, has revealed the measurable impact of nature on stress hormones. The cortisol levels that surge in response to life's demands find a subtle equilibrium in the serene embrace of green spaces. The symphony of nature, with its bird songs and rustling leaves, orchestrates a harmonious dance that resonates deep within us, calming the relentless cadence of stress.

In the heart of this chapter, we explore the physiological responses that occur when we immerse ourselves in the natural world. The calming effect on the nervous system, the reduction in cortisol production – these are not mere statistical notations but the silent language through which nature communicates with our bodies, offering a sanctuary of solace.

B. Outdoor Activities for Stress Relief

As we navigate the tumultuous waters of stress, we find ourselves drawn to the shores of outdoor activities that offer not only diversion but a profound sense of relief. Nature becomes the canvas upon which we paint our stress-free moments, each stroke a testament to the therapeutic potential of the great outdoors.

Hiking along a forest trail, the rhythmic crunch of leaves beneath our boots becomes a cadence that drowns out the cacophony of worries. The crisp air, infused with the scents of pine and earth, becomes a tonic for the weary soul. Science corroborates what our senses intuitively understand – outdoor activities are not just leisure pursuits; they are therapeutic interventions that recalibrate the mind and body.

In the company of flowing rivers or beneath the sheltering canopy of trees, we discover the transformative power of movement. Whether it's the steady rhythm of a kayak paddle slicing through still waters or the gentle swaying of a hammock suspended between two trees, outdoor activities become a conduit for stress relief. The very act of engaging with nature in motion becomes a meditation, a moving mindfulness that untangles the knots of stress one step, one paddle, one breath at a time.

C. Creating Tranquil Outdoor Spaces

In the tapestry of our lives, the spaces we inhabit hold the potential to either magnify or alleviate stress. As we venture into the art of creating tranquil outdoor spaces, we recognize that nature's role in stress reduction extends beyond the boundaries of wilderness. It is a presence that can be woven into the fabric of our everyday environments.

A tranquil outdoor space need not be grandiose; it is a testament to intentionality and simplicity. In the nooks of urban landscapes or the corners of suburban gardens, we discover the capacity to cultivate oases of calm. A small patio adorned with potted plants, a balcony overlooking a city skyline, or a secluded reading nook beneath the branches of a shade tree – these are the canvases upon which we paint tranquility.

Scientifically, the impact of these outdoor sanctuaries on stress reduction is profound. Blood pressure lowers, heart rates steady, and the mind finds reprieve from the relentless chatter. Yet, beyond the scientific metrics, there is an innate understanding that these tranquil outdoor spaces are the vessels through which nature's healing energy flows into our lives.

In the concluding verses of this chapter, we find ourselves surrounded by the tangible and intangible threads of stress reduction that nature weaves. The impact on stress hormones, the therapeutic dance of outdoor activities, and the creation of tranquil outdoor spaces - each thread contributes to the symphony of well-being.

As we stand at the crossroads of stress and serenity, let us linger in the knowledge that nature, with its quiet wisdom, holds the keys to unlocking the gates of tranquility. In the chapters that follow, we shall continue our exploration, delving into the nuances of nature's role in our holistic well-being. But for now, let us revel in the gentle breeze, the rustling leaves, and the quiet spaces where stress unravels and serenity blossoms.

5

The Verdant Prescription: Nature's Gift to Physical Well-Being

A. Immune System Boost through Nature Exposure

In the dance of seasons and the whisper of leaves, nature extends a subtle invitation to bolster our immune systems through exposure to its myriad wonders. This chapter unfurls the pages of a verdant prescription, exploring the immune system boost that accompanies our communion with the natural world.

Science, akin to a diligent gardener, tends to the empirical evidence that reveals the impact of nature exposure on our immune function. The phytoncides released by trees, the aromatic compounds that waft through the air in forests – these are not mere olfactory pleasures but agents that fortify our immune defenses. As we inhale the essence of the natural world, our bodies respond with an increased production of white blood cells and a bolstering of immune activity.

The intricate dance between nature and our immune systems is not a recent revelation; it is a dialogue that has echoed through the ages. From the healing groves of ancient civilizations to the modern green prescriptions endorsed by healthcare professionals, the link between nature and immune health is a perennial thread that weaves through the fabric of our existence.

B. Exercise and Healing in Natural Environments

As we tread the verdant pathways that wind through meadows and mountains, we unearth the symbiotic relationship between exercise, healing, and natural environments. Nature becomes not just a backdrop for physical activity but an active participant in the regenerative processes that unfold within our bodies.

In the embrace of outdoor spaces, we find the canvas upon which exercise becomes a transformative journey. Whether it's the rhythmic cadence of a trail run, the meditative flow of yoga beneath a canopy of trees, or the invigorating splash of waves during a coastal swim, exercise in nature transcends the boundaries of routine. The healing energy of the natural world infuses each movement, each breath, with a vitality that transcends the confines of gym walls.

Scientifically, the benefits of exercise in natural settings are manifold. The cardiovascular system is invigorated, stress hormones are reduced, and the mind experiences a clarity that is often elusive within indoor environments. Yet, beyond the scientific metrics, there is a profound understanding that nature's contribution to physical well-being extends beyond the quantifiable. It is an alchemy that transforms exercise into a holistic and rejuvenating experience.

C. Nature's Contribution to Faster Recovery

In the delicate tapestry of recovery, nature emerges as an invaluable ally, contributing to the swifter healing of body and mind. This chapter unfurls the pages of stories that speak to nature's role in expediting recovery, whether from illness, surgery, or the weariness of life's demands.

Scientific studies, akin to gentle rain on a parched landscape, reveal the measurable impact of natural settings on the recovery process.

Patients in hospital rooms with views of green spaces experience faster recovery times, reduced pain medication requirements, and a more positive outlook. Nature becomes the unspoken companion in the healing journey, its presence a balm that accelerates the restoration of health.

Beyond the confines of hospital walls, we encounter narratives of individuals who have embraced nature as a partner in their recovery. From coastal walks that breathe life into weary lungs to mountain retreats that rejuvenate the spirit, the stories affirm that nature's contribution to faster recovery is not confined to medical settings. It is an ever-present force that whispers healing into the spaces where we tread.

As we conclude this chapter, we stand amidst the vibrant hues of nature's physical health benefits, a tapestry woven with threads of immune resilience, exercise vitality, and accelerated recovery. In the chapters that follow, we shall journey deeper into the realms where nature's touch continues to unfold its layers of well-being. For now, let us revel in the knowledge that the verdant prescription for physical health is not merely a remedy; it is a timeless gift bestowed upon us by the healing embrace of the natural world.

6

Whispers of the Soul: Nature's Tender Embrace for Mental and Emotional Well-Being

A. Nature's Effect on Mental Health Disorders

In the sanctuary of rustling leaves and the gentle cadence of flowing waters, we uncover the profound impact of nature on mental health disorders. This chapter is an exploration of the healing dance between the natural world and the complexities of our minds – a journey where the sun-dappled paths of ancient forests become a refuge for the soul.

Scientific studies, much like the intricate patterns etched on a leaf, unfold the evidence of nature's effect on mental health. From anxiety to depression, nature emerges as a quiet but formidable ally in the quest for emotional well-being. Time spent in green spaces has been linked to a reduction in symptoms associated with mental health disorders, and the therapeutic potential of natural settings is increasingly recognized by clinicians and researchers alike.

As we meander through the research, we find stories of individuals who have sought solace in the embrace of nature amidst the tumult of their mental health journeys. The green therapy of woodland walks, the gentle hum of a forest clearing, or the serene vista of a mountain summit – these are not merely anecdotal tales but testimonials to the transformative power of nature in healing the mind.

B. Emotional Resilience and Nature Connection

In the fragile tapestry of our emotions, nature becomes both anchor and guide, fostering emotional resilience through a profound connection that transcends the tangible and enters the realm of the soul. This chapter unravels the threads of emotional resilience that nature weaves, exploring the ways in which our connection to the natural world fortifies our inner landscapes.

The concept of emotional resilience is not about avoiding the storms of life but about learning to dance in the rain. Nature becomes the gentle instructor, revealing that strength is not found in unyielding rigidity but in the flexible sway of grasses beneath the wind. As we cultivate a deeper connection with the natural world, we discover that our emotional resilience is nurtured by the rhythms of nature – the cycles of growth, the seasons of change, and the constant renewal that defines the natural order.

Through the lens of emotional resilience, we witness the stories of those who have found refuge in the embrace of nature during times of emotional upheaval. From the cathartic release of tears on a deserted beach to the quiet contemplation amidst the grandeur of a mountain range, these stories affirm that nature's role in emotional well-being is not just about joyous moments but about providing a safe haven for our most vulnerable selves.

C. Therapeutic Practices Integrating Nature

The therapeutic alliance between nature and mental and emotional well-being extends beyond happenstance encounters. In this chapter, we delve into intentional practices that seamlessly weave nature into therapeutic interventions, creating a holistic approach that recognizes the profound impact of the natural world on our psychological landscapes.

Ecotherapy, forest bathing, and nature-based counseling emerge as therapeutic practices that integrate nature into the healing journey. These approaches acknowledge that mental and emotional well-being is not confined to the walls of a counseling room but is intricately linked to the landscapes that surround us. In the quiet spaces of a woodland retreat or the serenity of a natural sanctuary, individuals find a canvas upon which their stories can unfold, and healing can commence.

The therapeutic practices are not prescriptions to be followed rigorously but invitations to engage with nature as a co-facilitator in the therapeutic process. Whether it's the meditative stillness of a forest meditation or the expressive freedom of art therapy amidst nature's canvas, these practices affirm that the natural world is not just a backdrop to therapy but an active participant in the transformative journey towards mental and emotional well-being.

In the concluding verses of this chapter, we stand amidst the nuanced beauty of nature's impact on our mental and emotional well-being. The whispers of the soul that echo through the rustling leaves, the emotional resilience cultivated in the quiet embrace of nature, and the intentional therapeutic practices that seamlessly integrate the natural world into our healing journeys – these are the threads that weave the intricate tapestry of well-being.

As we turn the pages towards the chapters that follow, let us carry with us the profound understanding that nature is not just a healer of ailments but a tender companion in the realms of our minds and hearts. In the chapters that follow, we shall continue our exploration, navigating the landscapes where nature's touch continues to unfold its layers of well-being. For now, let us linger in the tranquil spaces where the soul finds solace amidst the branches, and the heart resonates with the gentle hum of the natural world.

7

Nature's Palette: A Source of Inspiration for the Creative Soul

A. Creativity and Nature Connection

In the dappled sunlight filtering through leaves, the rustling of branches, and the symphony of birdsong, we uncover the wellspring of creativity that flows from the intimate connection between artists and the natural world. This chapter embarks on a journey through the boundless realms where creativity and nature converge, exploring the ways in which the great outdoors becomes both muse and mentor to the creative spirit.

Creativity, like the blooming of wildflowers in a meadow, flourishes when it is rooted in a connection to nature. This is not a mere romantic notion but a sentiment echoed through the annals of artistic history and validated by the whispers of countless creators. In the embrace of nature, artists find inspiration that transcends the limitations of the studio, writers unearth narratives woven into the landscape, and innovators glimpse solutions that emerge from the patterns of the natural world.

As we immerse ourselves in the connection between creativity and nature, we find that the act of creation becomes a dance with the elements. Whether it's the strokes of a paintbrush capturing the play of light on leaves or the rhythmic tapping of keys transcribing the cadence of a flowing river, the creative process becomes a dialogue with nature. Through this communion, artists discover that the well of inspiration is not a finite reservoir but an ever-flowing stream that meanders through the landscapes of their imagination.

B. Stories of Artists, Writers, and Innovators Inspired by Nature

The pages of artistic history are illuminated by the stories of creators who have forged profound connections with the natural world, drawing inspiration from its beauty, complexity, and inherent narratives. In this chapter, we unravel the tales of artists, writers, and innovators whose works have been shaped by the indelible mark of nature's inspiration.

Among the verdant hills of the Hudson Valley, we encounter the story of the Hudson River School painters – a group of 19th-century artists who found their muse in the American landscape. The grandeur of nature, from the sweeping vistas to the intricate details, became a canvas upon which they painted not just scenes but emotions and narratives. The Hudson River School is a testament to the transformative power of nature to elevate art beyond mere representation to a realm where the spirit of the land is captured on canvas.

In the quietude of a lakeside cabin, we find the footprints of writers like Henry David Thoreau, whose transcendental prose emerged from his communion with Walden Pond. The simple act of observing nature became a gateway to philosophical reflections, and the solitude of the woods became the crucible for literary masterpieces. Thoreau's stories resonate with the understanding that nature is not just a backdrop but a collaborator in the creative process.

In the chapters of technological innovation, we uncover the footprints of innovators who drew inspiration from the intricacies of the natural world. Biomimicry, the practice of emulating nature's designs and processes in human inventions, reveals the symbiotic relationship between innovation and nature. From Velcro inspired by burdock burrs to high-efficiency wind turbines modeled after humpback whale flippers, these stories affirm that nature is not just a source of artistic inspiration but a wellspring of inventive ideas.

C. Techniques for Tapping into Nature's Creative Energy

For those seeking to tap into nature's creative energy, this chapter offers a guide to intentional practices that nurture the symbiotic relationship between creativity and the natural world. These techniques are not rigid formulas but invitations to engage with nature as a co-creator in the creative process.

Nature journaling, a practice that involves recording observations, sketches, and reflections during outdoor experiences, becomes a gateway to tapping into nature's creative energy. Whether seated beneath the shade of a tree or perched on a rock overlooking a canyon, the act of journaling becomes a dialogue with the landscape, capturing not just images but the essence of the moment.

Similarly, the practice of plein air painting invites artists to set up their easels outdoors, capturing the changing light and colors of nature in real-time. The canvas becomes a portal through which the artist translates the energy of the landscape onto the painting, and the act of creation becomes a dynamic exchange between the artist and nature.

For writers, the practice of nature writing becomes a conduit for tapping into the creative energy of the natural world. Whether crafting poetry amidst wildflowers or penning prose beneath the canopy of ancient trees, nature writing is an exploration of language that seeks to convey not just the visual aspects of the landscape but the emotions and stories embedded within it.

In the closing verses of this chapter, we stand amidst the vibrant hues of nature's inspiration for the creative soul. From the strokes of the paintbrush to the eloquence of the written word, the stories of artists, writers, and innovators affirm that nature is not just a muse but a profound collaborator in the act of creation.

As we turn the pages towards the chapters that follow, let us carry with us the understanding that nature's inspiration is not a fleeting muse but an enduring presence that enriches the creative spirit. In the chapters that follow, we shall continue our exploration, navigating the landscapes where creativity blossoms amidst the branches, and the imagination expands through our connection with nature.

8

Gardens of Solace: Cultivating Healing Spaces in a Concrete World

A. Design Principles for Therapeutic Gardens

In the gentle rustle of leaves and the fragrance of blooming flowers, healing gardens emerge as sanctuaries for the weary soul. This chapter invites us to stroll through the carefully designed landscapes where the principles of therapeutic gardening unfold, creating spaces that not only delight the senses but nurture well-being on a profound level.

Therapeutic gardens are not mere patches of greenery; they are intentional creations, designed with a deep understanding of how the natural world interacts with our senses and emotions. Amidst the soft textures of foliage, the vibrant colors of blossoms, and the soothing sounds of trickling water, these gardens become a tapestry woven with the threads of healing.

The principles guiding the design of therapeutic gardens are rooted in the recognition that nature has the power to evoke positive physiological and psychological responses. Elements such as curved pathways that meander like a gentle stream, sensory plantings that engage touch and scent, and quiet corners for reflection all contribute to the therapeutic experience.

As we wander through the lush contours of these healing spaces, we encounter the wisdom of designers who have seamlessly blended form and function. The inclusion of seating areas bathed in dappled sunlight, the strategic use of water features that mimic the calming sounds of nature, and the incorporation of native plants that resonate with a sense of place – each design element becomes a brushstroke in the canvas of therapeutic gardens.

B. Community Initiatives for Green Spaces

In the heart of bustling urban landscapes, community initiatives bloom like resilient wildflowers, advocating for and cultivating green spaces that serve as communal sanctuaries. This chapter unfolds the stories of these initiatives, where the collective spirit of communities comes together to transform neglected corners into vibrant oases of respite.

Community gardens, pocket parks, and urban green spaces are not just amenities; they are expressions of the collective desire for well-being in the heart of concrete jungles. Through grassroots efforts and collaborative endeavors, communities reclaim spaces that were once neglected, transforming them into havens where the rhythms of nature synchronize with the rhythms of community life.

In the heart of a bustling neighborhood, we find the story of a community garden that emerged from the shared vision of residents. What was once an abandoned lot now blossoms with raised beds of vegetables, flower borders that attract pollinators, and communal spaces where residents gather to cultivate not just plants but connections. The community garden becomes a living testament to the transformative power of collective stewardship over green spaces.

Similarly, pocket parks become vibrant hubs of activity and connection. Tucked between buildings or nestled in the midst of city blocks, these small oases offer a reprieve from the urban hustle. Whether it's a lunch break spent on a park bench or a community yoga class beneath the shade of a tree, these green pockets become the lungs of the city, breathing life into the spaces where people live, work, and play.

C. Accessible Nature for Urban Dwellers

For those navigating the urban labyrinth, the accessibility of nature becomes a crucial factor in the quest for well-being. This chapter illuminates the initiatives and innovations that bridge the gap between urban life and the restorative power of nature, ensuring that even in the heart of the city, accessible green spaces abound.

Urban planning and design, when infused with a commitment to accessible nature, become catalysts for positive change. The creation of green corridors, the integration of rooftop gardens, and the transformation of vacant lots into micro-parks all contribute to the weaving of nature into the fabric of urban living. These initiatives are not just about aesthetics but about recognizing the fundamental human need for connection with the natural world.

As we wander through the urban landscapes where accessible nature unfolds, we encounter stories of innovation that transcend the limitations of space. Rooftop gardens, suspended between the skyline and the sky, become elevated sanctuaries where urban dwellers can escape the confines of concrete and steel. Green roofs not only provide insulation and stormwater management but also offer spaces for respite and reflection.

The concept of biophilic design, which integrates natural elements into the built environment, becomes a guiding principle for architects and urban planners. From office buildings adorned with living walls to public spaces infused with the sounds of water features, biophilic design becomes a silent advocate for the seamless integration of nature into the urban experience.

In the concluding verses of this chapter, we find ourselves amidst the verdant landscapes of healing gardens and accessible green spaces.

The design principles that guide therapeutic gardens, the community initiatives that transform urban corners into havens, and the innovative approaches that bring nature within reach of urban dwellers – these are the layers of a narrative that speaks to the enduring human desire for connection with the natural world.

As we turn the pages towards the chapters that follow, let us carry with us the understanding that healing gardens and green spaces are not just aesthetic luxuries but essential components of our well-being. In the chapters that follow, we shall continue our exploration, navigating the landscapes where nature's healing touch unfolds amidst the cityscape.

9

Nature's Daily Alchemy: Infusing Well-being into Modern Life

A. Practical Tips for Embracing Nature Daily

In the tapestry of modern life, where the demands of screens and schedules often drown out the whispers of the natural world, this chapter becomes a guidebook for weaving nature's healing touch into the fabric of our daily existence. Here, we embark on a journey of practical tips, exploring ways to infuse the balm of nature into our everyday routines.

The morning sun, with its golden glow, becomes a gentle beckoning to start our day with a moment of connection. Practical tip one: Begin your morning with a few minutes outdoors, whether it's a stroll in a nearby park, a pause on the balcony, or simply standing in the backyard with a cup of tea. This small ritual sets the tone for the day, grounding us in the rhythms of nature before the clamor of daily life takes center stage.

As we navigate the chapters of our day, practical tip two becomes a reminder to bring a bit of nature indoors. Whether it's placing a potted plant on the windowsill, arranging fresh flowers on the desk, or incorporating natural elements into home decor, these small gestures infuse our indoor spaces with the vitality of the outdoors. The subtle presence of nature becomes a constant companion, a reminder that even in the midst of urbanity, a touch of greenery can transform our surroundings.

Lunchtime, often relegated to hurried bites at the desk, becomes an opportunity for practical tip three: Take your lunch outdoors. Whether it's a nearby park, a quiet bench in a courtyard, or a green space near your workplace, stepping into nature during the lunch break becomes a pause that rejuvenates the mind and nourishes the body. The simple act of eating amidst the rustle of leaves or the hum of a city park becomes a culinary communion with the natural world.

The evening hours, as the day gently transitions into night, offer practical tip four: Embrace the golden hour. Whether it's a leisurely walk as the sun sets, a moment of reflection in the garden, or simply gazing at the changing hues of the sky, the golden hour becomes a daily ritual that aligns us with the natural rhythms of twilight. This small window of time becomes a bridge between the busyness of the day and the serenity of the night.

B. Balancing Technology and Nature Engagement

In the era of screens and digital connectivity, the delicate dance between technology and nature becomes a crucial consideration for well-being. This chapter explores the art of balancing the demands of the digital world with the restorative qualities of nature, recognizing that harmony between the two is essential for a holistic and balanced life.

Practical tip five: Establish tech-free zones in your daily routine. Whether it's the first hour after waking or the last hour before bedtime, designate spaces in your day where screens are set aside, and nature takes center stage. This intentional separation creates moments of respite, allowing the mind to recalibrate and the senses to engage with the natural world.

As we navigate the realms of work and technology, practical tip six becomes a reminder to incorporate nature into our virtual spaces. Whether it's setting nature-themed wallpapers on screens, joining virtual meetings from a balcony or garden, or incorporating nature sounds into the digital background, these small adjustments infuse our tech-centric world with the soothing presence of nature.

Practical tip seven invites us to engage with technology in ways that deepen our connection to the natural world. Whether it's using apps that identify bird calls, joining virtual nature communities, or participating in online gardening forums, technology becomes a tool for enhancing our understanding and appreciation of nature. It becomes a bridge that connects us to a global community of nature enthusiasts and experts.

C. Small Changes, Big Impact on Well-being

In the quiet corners of our daily routines, small changes become potent catalysts for well-being. This chapter unfolds the narrative of practical tips that, when embraced with intentionality, have the power to create a profound impact on our physical, mental, and emotional health.

Practical tip eight becomes an exploration of mindful moments in nature. Whether it's practicing mindful walking during a lunchtime stroll, engaging in nature-inspired breathing exercises, or simply pausing to observe the changing sky, these small moments of mindfulness become anchors that tether us to the present and infuse our lives with a sense of calm.

In the realm of self-care, practical tip nine invites us to integrate nature into our wellness routines. Whether it's incorporating natural elements into skincare rituals, practicing yoga in a park, or simply taking a moment to lie on the grass and gaze at the clouds, these small self-care rituals become acts of self-love infused with the healing energy of nature.

Practical tip ten becomes an invitation to cultivate a nature-inspired bedtime routine. Whether it's reading a few pages of a nature-themed book, listening to the sounds of a forest as you drift off to sleep, or simply gazing at the stars from your window, these small adjustments become a nightly ritual that nurtures restful sleep and sweet dreams.

In the concluding verses of this chapter, we find ourselves amidst the tapestry of practical tips that seamlessly integrate nature healing into our daily lives. From morning rituals that align us with the dawn to evening practices that usher in the night, each tip becomes a thread in the fabric of a life where nature is not a separate entity but an integral part of our well-being.

10

The Green Prescription: Nature's Therapeutic Touch

A. Overview of Ecotherapy and Forest Bathing

In the quiet spaces where leaves whisper and streams murmur, nature-based therapies unfold as gentle prescriptions for the soul. This chapter invites us into the verdant realms of ecotherapy and forest bathing, exploring the profound impact of intentional nature engagement on our holistic well-being.

Ecotherapy, much like a skilled herbalist crafting a remedy, encompasses a range of therapeutic practices that integrate nature into the healing process. Whether it's horticultural therapy, wilderness therapy, or nature-based counseling, ecotherapy recognizes the symbiotic relationship between the natural world and our psychological well-being. In the heart of community gardens, the tranquility of wooded trails, and the intentional use of natural elements in therapeutic settings, ecotherapy becomes a tapestry woven with threads of connection, healing, and growth.

Forest bathing, a practice rooted in ancient Japanese traditions, unfolds as a meditative communion with the forest. The act of immersing oneself in the sights, sounds, and scents of the forest becomes not just a leisurely stroll but a therapeutic endeavor that rejuvenates the mind, body, and spirit. The forest, with its towering trees and dappled sunlight, becomes a sanctuary where stress unravels, and well-being blossoms.

B. Guided Nature Meditations and Practices

In the hush of a quiet glade or the stillness of a mountain summit, guided nature meditations and practices become portals into the serene landscapes of our inner selves. This chapter becomes a guidebook for those seeking to harness the transformative power of intentional mindfulness amidst the embrace of the natural world.

Guided nature meditations invite us to attune our senses to the subtle symphony of the outdoors. Whether it's a meditation that focuses on the rhythmic cadence of ocean waves, the gentle rustle of leaves, or the chorus of birdsong, guided nature meditations become a voyage into the present moment. The act of grounding ourselves in the sensory delights of nature becomes a mindfulness practice that not only calms the mind but opens the door to a deeper connection with the environment.

Practical tip eleven: Incorporate nature-inspired mindfulness into your daily routine. Whether it's practicing mindful breathing beneath the canopy of trees, engaging in a walking meditation along a nature trail, or simply sitting in quiet contemplation in a garden, these small but intentional practices become seeds that sprout into a garden of tranquility within.

Beyond meditation, the practices extend to mindful engagement with the elements. Whether it's the practice of shinrin-yoku, or "forest bathing," where one immerses oneself in the sensory experiences of the forest, or the act of mindful observation of natural patterns and cycles, these practices become gateways to a heightened awareness that transcends the hurried pace of modern life.

C. Professional Guidance for Nature-Based Healing

In the hands of skilled guides and professionals, nature-based healing unfolds as a nuanced and intentional therapeutic modality. This chapter delves into the role of trained practitioners who shepherd individuals through the landscapes of nature-based therapies, offering expertise and support on the journey toward well-being.

The ecotherapist, much like a seasoned trailblazer, guides individuals on a journey of self-discovery through the natural world. Through a combination of outdoor activities, reflective practices, and intentional engagement with nature, ecotherapists become companions on the path to healing. Whether it's a therapeutic garden, a wilderness retreat, or the quietude of a natural sanctuary, the ecotherapist curates experiences that nurture resilience, foster growth, and kindle the innate healing capacities within.

Forest therapy guides, with the finesse of forest nymphs, lead individuals through the art of forest bathing. Trained to facilitate immersive nature experiences, forest therapy guides create a container for participants to engage with the forest in a mindful and intentional way. Through guided invitations, reflective prompts, and group sharing, these guides orchestrate forest bathing sessions that transcend the boundaries of a mere walk in the woods and become transformative journeys into the heart of nature.

Practical tip twelve: Seek professional guidance for nature-based healing when needed. Whether it's connecting with an ecotherapist, participating in a forest bathing session led by a certified guide, or engaging in nature-based counseling, seeking the expertise of trained professionals ensures that the healing journey is navigated with care, skill, and an understanding of the intricate interplay between nature and well-being.

In the concluding verses of this chapter, we stand at the crossroads of nature-based therapies, where ecotherapy and forest bathing converge as powerful avenues for healing. Guided by skilled professionals and practitioners, individuals find solace, renewal, and transformation in the embrace of the natural world.

As we turn the pages towards the chapters that follow, let us carry with us the understanding that nature-based therapies are not just interventions; they are profound invitations to commune with the healing energies of the earth. In the chapters that follow, we shall continue our exploration, navigating the landscapes where nature's therapeutic touch continues to unfold, and the inner self becomes grounded through our connections to nature.

11

Nature's Embrace: A Healing Symphony for the Soul

A. Recap of Nature's Healing Attributes

As we stand amidst the verdant tapestry woven by nature-based therapies, it is essential to recap the resplendent attributes that make the natural world an unparalleled healer of the human spirit. From the therapeutic embrace of ecotherapy to the meditative communion of forest bathing, nature's healing attributes unfold as a symphony that resonates with the core of our being.

The rhythm of leaves dancing in the wind, the melodic trickle of a babbling brook, and the symphony of birdsong that serenades the dawn – these are not merely auditory sensations but threads in the healing fabric of nature. The scientifically proven benefits of reduced stress, improved mood, and enhanced overall well-being become harmonious chords in the composition of nature's therapeutic song.

Ecotherapy, with its intentional fusion of outdoor activities, reflective practices, and communal engagement with nature, emerges as a holistic healer that tends to the mind, body, and spirit. Therapeutic gardens become sanctuaries where growth and resilience are nurtured, and forest bathing becomes a meditative journey that restores balance to the restless mind.

As we recap nature's healing attributes, let us not forget the timeless wisdom of indigenous cultures and the profound understanding that nature is not merely a backdrop but a wise and compassionate guide on the journey toward well-being. The principles of biophilia, the recognition of our innate connection to the natural world, echo through the chapters of nature-based therapies, affirming that our well-being is intricately woven into the ecosystems that cradle us.

B. Encouragement for Readers to Embrace Nature

In the gentle cadence of leaves and the fragrance of blossoms, there lies an invitation – a call to embrace nature as a steadfast companion on the path to well-being. This chapter resonates with the encouragement for readers to open their hearts to the healing touch of the natural world, to become active participants in the restorative dance between humanity and nature.

Practical tip thirteen: Embrace nature as a daily ritual. Whether it's a morning stroll in a local park, a mindful lunchtime pause in a green space, or an evening walk beneath the stars, make nature a regular part of your daily routine. Allow the sights, sounds, and scents of the outdoors to become familiar companions in the rhythm of your life.

As we navigate the demands of modernity, practical tip fourteen becomes a gentle reminder to cultivate a nature-inspired sanctuary in the home. Whether it's creating a small garden oasis on a balcony, incorporating natural elements into interior decor, or simply opening windows to invite in the freshness of the outdoors, these intentional acts become gestures of love that bridge the gap between the indoor and outdoor realms.

The encouragement extends to families and communities, practical tip fifteen calling for collective engagement with nature. Whether it's organizing community nature walks, establishing communal gardens, or advocating for green spaces in urban planning, these endeavors become expressions of shared stewardship over the landscapes that nurture us.

C. Call to Action for a Healthier, Nature-Connected Life

In the closing verses of this exploration into nature-based therapies, a resounding call to action emerges – a rallying cry for a healthier, nature-connected life. This chapter becomes a testament to the understanding that the pursuit of well-being is not a solitary endeavor but a collective movement toward a more harmonious relationship with the natural world.

Practical tip sixteen becomes a call to advocate for green initiatives in local communities. Whether it's supporting the creation of more therapeutic gardens, participating in tree-planting campaigns, or championing policies that prioritize access to green spaces, individuals become ambassadors for a healthier, nature-connected society.

As we turn the pages towards a future where nature and well-being are inseparable, practical tip seventeen becomes a reminder to share the wisdom of nature-based therapies with others. Whether it's recommending books on the subject, organizing workshops on ecotherapy, or simply engaging in conversations that highlight the healing power of nature, individuals become conduits for a ripple effect that extends far beyond the confines of personal well-being.

In the realms of education, practical tip eighteen becomes a call to integrate nature-based learning into curricula. Whether it's fostering outdoor classrooms, incorporating nature-inspired activities into lesson plans, or organizing field trips to natural spaces, educators become architects of an educational paradigm that recognizes nature as a potent teacher.

As we stand at the crossroads of a call to action for a healthier, nature-connected life, let us carry with us the understanding that our choices, both small and significant, have the power to shape a world where nature is not just a backdrop but an active participant in our collective well-being.

In the chapters that follow, let us embark on a journey where the healing touch of nature continues to unfold, where individuals become stewards of the land, and where communities resonate with the gentle hum of the natural world. For in the embrace of nature, we discover not just remedies for ailments but a timeless companion on the journey toward a life infused with well-being, vitality, and harmony.

12

Resources

Resources

Clinebell, H. (1996). Ecotherapy: Healing with Nature in Mind. San Francisco: Sierra Club Books.

Linden, S., & Grut, J. (2002). The Healing Fields: Working with Psychotherapy and Nature to Rebuild Shattered Lives. Frances Lincoln, London.

Kimmerer, R. W. (2013). Braiding Sweetgrass: Indigenous Wisdom, Scientific Knowledge, and the Teachings of Plants. Milkweed Editions.

Williams, F. (2017). The Nature Fix: Why Nature Makes Us Happier, Healthier, and More Creative. W. W. Norton & Company.